HOMESTEAD HEROES

Westerns for Seniors

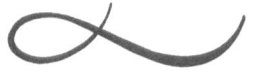

seniorality

Homestead Heroes -
Sam Suncroft
Copyright © 2024
Seniorality / Everbreeze Media Oy

This is a work of fiction. Names and characters are the product of the author's imagination and any resemblance to actual persons, living or dead, is entirely coincidental.

Set in EB Garamond

1. The New Deputy

The town of Sagebrush sat beneath a blazing sun, its streets quiet under the midday heat. Dust hung in the air, stirred only by the rare passing wagon or the occasional gust of wind. Today, however, there was a buzz among the few residents who dared venture out in the stifling heat. News had traveled fast—a new deputy had arrived, one said to be tough as nails and smart enough to outwit any outlaw this side of the Rockies.

James Hamilton rode slowly down the main road, taking in the empty storefronts and sun-baked buildings. His eyes were sharp beneath the brim of his worn hat, and his expression unreadable. He knew all too well that towns like this, clinging to life on the frontier, had their share of troubles.

Rustlers, gamblers, and drifters made their livings off the sweat and toil of honest folks who just wanted a bit of land to call their own. His gaze settled briefly on the saloon, then on the jail at the far end of town.

As he dismounted his horse and hitched it to a post outside the marshal's office, he caught sight of a few curious faces peeking out from windows. Sagebrush had seen its fair share of lawmen come and go, most unable or unwilling to stand up to Charles Jones and his band of enforcers. Jones ran a sprawling cattle operation to the west, and his reach extended far beyond his ranch. Everyone in Sagebrush knew better than to cross him, and those who didn't soon found out the hard way.

James opened the door to the marshal's office and stepped inside, greeted by the sight of Marshal Wyatt Jackson hunched over his desk, sorting through a stack of wanted posters. Jackson was older, with a gray beard and a weary look that suggested he'd spent too many years in this line of work.

"Deputy Hamilton," Jackson said, rising slowly and offering his hand. "Welcome to Sagebrush."

"Much obliged, Marshal," James replied, shaking the man's hand. He took a seat across from Jackson, removing his hat and setting it on his knee. "Heard you've been having a fair bit of trouble out here."

Jackson sighed, rubbing the back of his neck. "More than a fair bit, I'd say. We got rustlers thick as flies, and Charles Jones breathing down our necks at every turn. He owns half the cattle in this territory, and he's made it clear he won't let anyone stand in his way."

James nodded, his jaw tightening. He'd heard tales of men like Jones, men who thought the law was an inconvenience meant for others, not them. "I didn't come here to stand by and watch him run roughshod over the place," he said. "I intend to put a stop to it."

Jackson raised an eyebrow, almost amused. "You'd be the first. Jones has a way of getting what he wants, one way or another. Folks around here keep their heads down, don't ask questions. They know what happens to those who don't."

"I've dealt with men like him before," James replied evenly. "They're all the same, thinking they own everything they see. But they're just men, same as the rest of us. And sooner or later, they fall."

Jackson looked at him for a moment, as if sizing him up. "Well, you might just be the man for the job, Deputy. Just keep your wits about you. Jones has a lot of friends in high places, and he won't hesitate to send a message if he thinks someone's stepping out of line."

James tipped his hat and stood. "I'm counting on it, Marshal."

—-

Later that afternoon, James took a slow walk through the town, letting the residents get a look at him. He was aware of the whispers, the cautious glances from behind curtains and doors. Most of them were simply trying to survive, but there was a quiet, almost resigned fear in their faces, a weariness that told him they'd seen enough violence and loss.

Just as he was about to head back to the office, he caught sight of a woman leading a young girl down the dusty street. The woman was tall, her dark hair pinned neatly under a bonnet, and her expression was one of quiet determination. James noticed her clothing was plain but clean, the kind that spoke of hard work and pride. The little girl beside her clutched her hand, looking up at James with wide eyes.

The woman paused, meeting his gaze. She offered a slight nod in greeting, her eyes assessing but not unkind. "You must be the new deputy," she said, her voice steady.

"That's right," he replied, tipping his hat. "James Hamilton. And you are?"

"Abigail Kennedy," she said, introducing herself with a faint smile. "My daughter, Sarah." The little girl ducked behind her mother's skirt, peeking out with a shy curiosity.

"Ma'am," he replied, nodding to her and offering a smile to Sarah, who watched him intently, her young face still innocent and untouched by the hardships of the town.

Abigail's expression shifted slightly, as if weighing whether or not to say something more. "Things aren't easy out here, Deputy," she said finally. "Especially for folks like us."

James sensed there was more to her words than she was letting on. "I'm here to make them easier, Mrs. Kennedy. Starting with putting an end to the rustlers and anyone else causing trouble."

Her eyes lingered on him, almost as if searching for some assurance. "You're not the first to make promises like that," she said softly. "But I hope you'll be the one to keep them."

"I intend to," he replied. He held her gaze a moment longer before she nodded, turning to lead her daughter away.

As he watched them go, he felt a surge of resolve. There was something about Abigail Kennedy that spoke of quiet resilience, and he knew that she, like so many others, had likely suffered under Charles Jones's rule.

—-

That night, as the town settled into a restless slumber, James sat alone in the marshal's office, his hand resting on his revolver. The darkness outside was thick, the kind that had its own weight, pressing down on the land.

He knew that soon enough, Charles Jones would hear of his arrival, and he'd be ready to make a move.

James welcomed it. He'd faced men like Jones before—powerful, arrogant men who thought they owned everything they saw. He'd learned to be patient, to wait for the right moment. In time, Jones would come for him, and when he did, James would be ready.

The clock on the wall ticked softly in the silence, and outside, the wind stirred the dust on Sagebrush's empty streets. James leaned back in his chair, eyes narrowed as he thought of the challenges ahead. This wasn't just another job; it was a chance to stand up for the people of Sagebrush and make a difference.

And he was prepared to do whatever it took to bring justice to this town.

2. Trouble on the Homestead

James Hamilton had only been in Sagebrush for a few days when he heard the first rumors about trouble brewing on the outskirts of town. Folks in the saloon were tight-lipped, exchanging cautious glances when he walked in, but James had a way of picking up on conversations meant to stay hidden. A few offhand remarks, a name whispered in fear—Abigail Kennedy.

Later that afternoon, as he strolled past the livery, he caught sight of an older ranch hand tending to his horse. The man nodded respectfully, tipping his hat. James took it as an invitation to strike up a conversation.

"I hear there's been some trouble out at Mrs. Kennedy's homestead," he said, keeping his tone casual.

The ranch hand's expression shifted, a flicker of unease in his eyes. "I don't know nothin' about that, Deputy," he replied, though his hands tightened on the reins. "It's best not to meddle in things that don't concern ya."

"Trouble on anyone's land concerns me," James replied evenly. "Mrs. Kennedy doesn't strike me as the type to cause trouble. Who's giving her grief?"

The ranch hand hesitated, then glanced around as if someone might be listening. "Jones's men," he said quietly, almost a whisper. "Been after her land for months now. Folks say her property cuts through the best graze in these parts, a shortcut for Jones's cattle to reach the valley beyond."

James felt his jaw tighten. "Thanks for the information," he said, nodding at the man.

He knew well enough that Charles Jones wasn't the kind to give up on anything he set his sights on, and it seemed that Abigail's land was no exception.

—-

Early the next morning, James saddled his horse and set off toward Abigail Kennedy's homestead, the town disappearing behind him as he rode into the open prairie. The land was vast, stretching out under a bright sky with scrub grass and the occasional cluster of trees dotting the landscape. He could see why Jones would want this land. It was prime territory, with rolling hills that led down toward a shallow valley where grass grew thick and green.

As he approached the homestead, he saw signs of disturbance—a broken fence, churned-up dirt where hoofprints marked the ground. It didn't take a trained eye to see that cattle had been driven through her property, likely as a warning or to scare her into leaving.

He rode up to the small house, which stood against a backdrop of low hills. The place was modest, with a simple porch and a few sturdy wooden beams supporting a weather-worn roof. Abigail was outside, working near the barn, a rifle slung over her shoulder. She looked up as he approached, her expression guarded.

"Deputy Hamilton," she greeted him with a nod, her voice steady. "Didn't expect to see you out here."

James dismounted, giving her a respectful nod. "I heard there's been trouble," he said. "Thought I'd come by and see for myself."

She sighed, glancing at the broken fence line. "You could say that. I've had Jones's men on my land more than I care to count, driving cattle through my fields, trampling what little I have planted."

"Why does he want your land?" James asked, though he suspected he already knew.

Abigail looked off toward the horizon, her eyes hard. "This property cuts right through to the grazing land Jones wants. If he controlled it, he could move his cattle to the valley faster and avoid having to take the long way around." She shook her head, a faint bitterness in her voice. "This land was my husband's, God rest his soul. He worked hard for it, and I won't let some bully force me off it."

James felt a surge of respect for her resilience. She wasn't a woman who would give up easily, and he admired that. But he knew that Charles Jones wouldn't be discouraged by one woman standing her ground.

"Mind if I take a look around?" he asked, glancing toward the broken fence.

Abigail nodded, though he could see the flicker of worry in her eyes. "Suit yourself. They've been coming through at night mostly. I keep watch, but they're clever about it. By the time I hear anything, they're already gone."

James walked over to the fence, crouching to examine the posts. It was clear that the damage wasn't accidental. Several of the posts had been snapped, not worn down by time or weather, and hoofprints were scattered around, suggesting the cattle had been herded deliberately.

He straightened, turning back to Abigail. "I'll make sure this stops," he said firmly. "But I can't be here every night."

Abigail glanced at him, her expression softening just a bit. "I appreciate that, Deputy. But you don't need to get mixed up in my troubles. Folks here know better than to stand up to Jones."

"I'm not most folks," he replied, his voice steady. "Jones needs to know there's law here now, and that it applies to him as well."

She gave him a long look, as if weighing his words. Finally, she nodded. "Then I suppose I'm in your debt."

James nodded and mounted his horse. "I'll be back tomorrow to check in," he promised. "In the meantime, stay alert. Jones won't give up easily."

Abigail's lips quirked into a small, rueful smile. "He hasn't yet. But neither have I."

As James rode away, he couldn't shake the thought of her standing alone on her land, facing down Jones's men with nothing but a rifle and her own unyielding spirit. The prairie was a harsh place, and it favored the strong, but he had the sense that Abigail Kennedy was as strong as they came.

—-

That evening, back in Sagebrush, James met with Marshal Jackson in the dimly lit confines of the marshal's office. Jackson sat behind his desk, his face cast in shadow as he listened to James's report.

"It's as we suspected," James said. "Jones's men have been after Abigail's land, trying to scare her off. They're herding cattle through her fields, breaking her fences."

Jackson sighed, shaking his head. "She's a stubborn one, that Abigail. Been holding out on that land for years. But Jones won't stop until he gets what he wants."

"Then it's time we made it clear he won't get it," James replied, his voice firm.

Jackson gave him a cautious look. "Be careful, Deputy. Jones has half the town in his pocket. It won't do us any good if you end up buried on the prairie."

James met his gaze with quiet resolve. "I didn't come here to sit back and watch people like Jones run roughshod over decent folks. He'll know soon enough that there's a new lawman in town."

The marshal studied him for a moment, then nodded slowly. "All right, Hamilton. But keep your wits about you. Jones won't take kindly to being challenged."

As James left the office and walked out into the darkened street, he felt a chill settle over him, the weight of the task ahead heavy on his shoulders. He knew the battle was just beginning, and that Charles Jones wouldn't back down without a fight.

But he was ready.

3. The Cattle Stampede

The sun was just beginning to dip below the horizon when James Hamilton rode out along the edge of the Kennedy homestead. The sky burned with a deep orange glow, casting long shadows over the rolling plains and rugged hills. He'd made a habit of patrolling this area every evening, a silent promise to Abigail and the other settlers that someone was watching, that the law hadn't forgotten them.

He reined in his horse atop a small rise, taking in the expanse of land stretching out before him. The cattle tracks were clear, cutting through fields and skirting the edges of fences. Abigail wasn't the only one with land in Jones's path—several other homesteaders had been affected, their fields trampled and fences left in shambles. It was a pattern he was beginning to recognize.

Then he heard it—the low, ominous rumble of pounding hooves, rolling across the plains like distant thunder. His eyes narrowed as he scanned the horizon, spotting a faint cloud of dust rising in the distance, moving fast toward the nearby homesteads.

A stampede.

Without wasting a second, James spurred his horse forward, racing across the open land as the rumbling grew louder. He could see the cattle now, a massive, seething mass of animals being driven straight toward the homesteads. And behind them, riding hard and pushing them forward, were a handful of riders he recognized all too well—Jones's men, spurring the cattle onward, knowing the destruction they would cause.

The riders had set the stampede in motion, and it was aimed directly at the carefully tended fields and fences of the homesteaders who had refused to sell to Jones.

James grit his teeth, pushing his horse to the limit. If he could get ahead of the cattle, maybe he could divert them away from the worst of it. But the herd was enormous, a dark, churning wave of horns and hooves tearing through the land with unstoppable force. He could already see fences shattering under the onslaught, fields reduced to trampled earth.

As he rode alongside the stampede, James caught sight of one of the homesteaders—a man named Hank Miller—scrambling to save his livestock. Hank's eyes widened as he saw James riding hard toward him.

"Hank!" James shouted over the deafening roar of hooves. "Get your family inside! Lock the doors and stay put!"

Hank didn't need to be told twice. He waved his thanks and took off toward his small house in the distance, disappearing into the dusk as the stampede bore down on them.

James urged his horse ahead, trying to find some way to divert the massive herd. The riders at the rear of the stampede spotted him, and he saw one of them—Clayton Yates, Jones's most trusted enforcer—sneer and raise his hat in a mocking salute.

James's jaw clenched, fury sparking in his chest. Yates and his men were riding hard to keep the cattle moving, deliberately sending them into the homestead lands. They weren't just rustlers—they were saboteurs, using the herd as a weapon, knowing that no farmer could withstand such destruction.

With no other choice, James angled his horse to intercept the cattle, drawing his revolver and firing shots into the air. The crack of gunfire echoed across the plains, startling the lead animals. A few of them veered off, but the mass of the herd kept moving forward, their panic too deeply set. The thunder of their hooves filled the air, drowning out even the gunshots.

James's horse bucked beneath him, nervous and frantic, but he kept a steady hand on the reins, urging it onward. He had to get closer—had to do something, anything to break the momentum of the herd.

But the stampede surged on, relentless. He barely managed to keep his horse steady as the animals pressed in on him, the ground shaking beneath the force of hundreds of pounding hooves. Dust filled his lungs, and the cacophony of bellowing cattle and snapping fence posts created a wall of noise that was almost overpowering.

Then he saw Abigail's homestead in the distance, her small house silhouetted against the darkening sky. His heart lurched. If the stampede reached her property, her fields would be obliterated, and her home might not even survive the impact.

He spurred his horse with a renewed urgency, trying to ride ahead of the herd, but it was like fighting against a raging river. He could see Abigail and her daughter on the porch, Abigail's face taut with fear as she watched the approaching chaos. Sarah, her young daughter, clung to her mother's side, wide-eyed.

"Get inside!" James shouted as he passed by, his voice barely carrying over the roar of the stampede. Abigail scooped Sarah into her arms and disappeared into the house, slamming the door shut just as the herd came crashing over her fence line.

James knew he couldn't stop the herd, but he could try to guide it away from the house. He fired several more shots into the air, steering his horse close to the edges of the stampede, trying to push the animals in a different direction. A few turned, veering away from the homestead, but it was only a fraction of the herd. The rest continued forward, drawn by their own blind terror.

A flash of movement caught his eye, and he realized that Yates and one of the other riders were bearing down on him, their faces hard with malice. They were coming after him, using the stampede as cover to try and take him out.

James tightened his grip on the reins, gritting his teeth as he realized he was caught between the stampede and Jones's men. He could either try to outrun the herd or face off with Yates. Neither option was good, but he didn't have time to hesitate.

With a swift kick, he urged his horse to the side, veering away from the main body of the stampede. Yates was right behind him, close enough now that James could see the glint of metal in his hand. A gunshot rang out, the sound sharp and deadly against the backdrop of chaos.

James ducked low, feeling the bullet whip past his shoulder. He twisted in the saddle, aiming his revolver and firing back. Yates dodged, swearing under his breath as he pulled his horse sharply to the side. But the other rider wasn't as lucky—James's shot found its mark, and the man toppled from his horse, disappearing into the dust.

Yates snarled and pulled back, his expression dark as he reined his horse away from James. But he wasn't retreating. He was regrouping, circling back with a deadly glint in his eye, ready to make another pass.

Just as Yates started to ride toward him again, James saw an opportunity. A narrow break in the stampede—a brief gap between the thronging animals that could allow him to cut through the herd and reach safer ground.

With a silent prayer, he spurred his horse forward, weaving through the stampede, dodging around the terrified cattle as they thundered past. It was like threading a needle, each step a gamble, but he managed to break through, emerging on the other side of the herd, his breath coming in short, sharp gasps.

When he turned to look back, he saw Yates and the remaining riders, but they had pulled up short, their silhouettes fading into the dust as the herd continued its relentless path.

James didn't stop until he reached a safe distance, watching as the stampede finally began to peter out, the remaining cattle scattering across the plains. His body ached, his pulse racing, but he'd managed to divert enough of the herd to spare the homesteads from complete devastation.

As the dust settled, he could see Abigail emerge from her house, her face filled with a mixture of relief and exhaustion. He gave her a nod, silently promising her that he would keep fighting, no matter how many stampedes Jones threw their way.

One way or another, he was going to bring Jones and his men to justice.

4. Meeting With the Marshal

James Hamilton strode through the dusty streets of Sagebrush, his mind still racing with the events of the stampede. The town bustled around him, with people going about their business, unaware—or perhaps choosing to ignore—the growing threat just outside their borders. But for James, ignoring it wasn't an option. He had seen firsthand the lengths to which Charles Jones was willing to go, and he knew that sooner or later, the violence would reach the town itself if no one stepped up to stop it.

His boots echoed on the wooden steps of the marshal's office as he approached the door, dust swirling in the late morning sunlight. The office was small and unassuming, a single-story building with a cracked window and peeling paint—a stark contrast to the sprawling, manicured ranch house that Jones called home. The town's marshal, Wyatt Jackson, was known as a fair man, but one whose loyalty sometimes swayed with the prevailing winds.

James opened the door, stepping into the dimly lit room. Jackson sat at his desk, his hat tipped low over his eyes, chewing on the end of an unlit cigar. He looked up as James entered, his expression a mixture of curiosity and apprehension.

"Deputy," Jackson greeted, nodding slightly. "I heard there was some trouble out on the Kennedy homestead last night."

James took a seat across from the marshal, placing his hat on his knee. "Trouble's putting it lightly," he replied, his voice grim. "Jones's men started a stampede, aimed it straight at the homesteads. They nearly tore down Abigail Kennedy's place, and they would've if I hadn't been there."

Jackson let out a low sigh, rubbing his temples. "Jones and his men have been a problem in these parts for years, Hamilton. You're not the first lawman to try to put him in his place."

"Then it's time someone did," James said firmly. "Jones has crossed a line, Marshal. I can't just stand by and let him keep terrorizing innocent people. If we don't stop him now, he's only going to get bolder."

Jackson leaned back in his chair, considering James with weary eyes. "You're a good man, Deputy. I don't doubt your heart's in the right place. But Jones...he's got a lot of influence in this town. Half the businesses in Sagebrush owe him money, and the other half are scared of him. You try to go up against him, you won't just be facing his men—you'll be fighting this whole town's way of life."

James's jaw tightened, frustration simmering beneath the surface. "So what are we supposed to do, Wyatt? Let him drive people off their land? Stand by while he destroys their property?"

Jackson sighed again, fiddling with the cigar between his fingers. "I don't like it any more than you do, Hamilton. But I've seen what happens when someone tries to take on Jones. They end up run out of town, or worse. This town's not ready to rise up against him, and you and I both know we don't have the manpower to take on his entire operation."

"We don't need an army," James argued, leaning forward. "We just need the law. If we start enforcing it—really enforcing it—people will see that Jones isn't above it. Maybe that's all it takes to give them the courage to stand up to him."

Jackson shook his head slowly. "I admire your idealism, Deputy. But people don't just change because someone tells them to. You go after Jones, and it's not just you he'll be coming for. He'll go after anyone who's close to you, anyone who stands with you. He's ruthless, and he's not afraid to make examples out of people."

James's expression hardened. "So what are you saying, Marshal? That we just let him run roughshod over the town? Over the people who are trying to make a life here?"

"I'm saying you have to pick your battles," Jackson replied, his tone cautious. "You can't take on every injustice, James. And sometimes, you have to accept that fighting a losing battle doesn't help anyone."

James stood up, his frustration boiling over. "With all due respect, Wyatt, this isn't a losing battle. It's a fight worth having. Maybe Jones has power now, but that doesn't make what he's doing right. If we don't stand up to him, who will?"

Jackson regarded him in silence for a long moment, his eyes searching James's face. Finally, he let out a weary sigh and leaned forward, placing his hands on the desk.

"Look, I don't want you to think I don't respect what you're trying to do," he said quietly. "But I've seen this before. Lawmen who come here with big ideas, thinking they can change things. And you know where they ended up?"

James waited, his gaze steady.

"Gone," Jackson said simply. "Or worse."

"Then maybe it's time someone saw it through," James replied, undeterred. "Maybe it's time this town remembered what it means to have a lawman who's not afraid to do his job."

Jackson hesitated, his gaze dropping to the desk as he considered James's words. For a moment, it looked as though he might be swayed. But then he shook his head, his face settling into a grim expression.

"You're a good man, James," he said finally. "But if you go after Jones, you're on your own. I can't risk the town's safety, or mine, by going toe-to-toe with him. Not unless you've got the townsfolk behind you."

James clenched his jaw, disappointment gnawing at him. "So that's it? You're just going to let him keep doing whatever he wants?"

Jackson's shoulders slumped. "I don't like it, but that's the reality of this place. This isn't the first time Jones has made trouble, and it won't be the last. Unless you find some way to turn the people against him, he'll just keep coming back, no matter what we do."

James took a deep breath, the bitter taste of helplessness filling his mouth. He'd hoped for more—hoped that the marshal would have the courage to stand up to Jones, even if it was risky. But he could see now that Jackson was too entrenched in the town's politics, too worn down by years of compromise.

Still, he wasn't ready to give up. "Fine," he said, his voice steady. "If you won't stand with me, I'll do it on my own. But know this, Marshal—if Jones brings trouble to this town, it'll be because we didn't stop him when we had the chance."

Jackson met his gaze, a flicker of regret passing over his face. "I hope you're wrong, Deputy. For all our sakes."

Without another word, James turned and walked out of the marshal's office, the door swinging shut behind him with a final, hollow thud. Outside, the town was bathed in golden light, but to James, it felt as though a shadow hung over everything, cast by the man who had twisted Sagebrush into his personal fiefdom.

As he walked down the main street, he caught sight of a few familiar faces—

townsfolk who nodded respectfully as he passed, others who avoided his gaze. He knew they were watching, waiting to see what he would do next. Jones had a hold over this town, but James was beginning to suspect that not everyone was as loyal to the cattle baron as they seemed. Perhaps, if he could rally the right people, he might stand a chance.

A flicker of determination sparked within him as he considered his options. He would need allies if he was going to make a stand against Jones—people with the courage to defy the status quo, people who believed that justice was worth the fight, no matter the cost.

He thought of Abigail, her fierce resolve and unwavering determination. He thought of Hank Miller, the rancher whose family had been nearly trampled by Jones's stampede. And he thought of the countless other settlers who had come to Sagebrush looking for a better life, only to find themselves caught in the web of fear and control that Jones had spun.

As he walked, his resolve hardened. He might be just one man, but he was a lawman, and that meant something. It had to mean something.

James Hamilton wasn't about to back down. Not now. Not ever.

5. Abigail's Plight

The Kennedy homestead sat nestled against the rising hills, its modest farmhouse surrounded by fields and a small garden. But where it should have felt like a sanctuary, the property instead bore scars from recent turmoil—broken fences, trampled soil, and a tension that hung in the air like a storm cloud. James could sense it the moment he approached the house.

He reined in his horse near the front porch and dismounted, tipping his hat as he caught sight of Abigail watching him from the doorway. She looked tired, her face drawn and her shoulders slumped. But there was a fire in her eyes, one that told him she was far from defeated.

"Deputy Hamilton," she greeted, attempting a weary smile. "Thank you for coming."

"Of course," he replied, stepping up onto the porch. "I wanted to check in on you, make sure you and Sarah were all right."

Abigail glanced back toward the house, where her young daughter was busy stacking blocks of wood near the fireplace. "We're managing," she said, her voice steady but tinged with exhaustion. "But I'd be lying if I said we weren't scared."

James's face softened. "I don't blame you. Jones and his men...they're relentless. And they know you're standing in the way of what he wants most."

Abigail nodded, crossing her arms as if to hold herself together. "It's not just the land," she murmured. "It's the way they look at us—like we're intruders. Like we have no right to be here."

Her words cut deep. James had seen that look many times—men like Jones and his crew, who believed their power gave them ownership over everything and everyone in their path. They were used to getting what they wanted, regardless of the cost.

"I know what it's like to feel that way," he said quietly, surprising himself with the admission. He rarely spoke of his past, the reasons that had driven him to take up the badge and leave everything else behind. But standing here with Abigail, he felt a connection—a shared understanding that needed no words.

She looked at him, curiosity mingling with empathy. "Do you?"

He took a deep breath, his gaze drifting over the landscape beyond her porch. "I lost my family to men like Jones. People who thought they could take whatever they wanted, regardless of the lives they ruined. It was a long time ago, but...some things don't leave you."

Abigail's expression softened, and she reached out, placing a gentle hand on his arm. "I'm sorry, James. I didn't know."

"It's all right," he replied, though his voice was rougher than he intended. "But it's why I can't just sit by and let Jones do this to you, or to anyone else here. I made a promise to myself that I'd never turn a blind eye again."

She nodded, her grip tightening slightly. "We're not giving up," she said fiercely, her voice trembling. "I won't let him take our home. Not after all we've been through to build it."

For a moment, they stood in silence, the weight of shared hardship hanging between them. He admired her strength, the quiet resilience that kept her rooted to this land despite the dangers. She was more than a match for Jones's threats, but no one should have to face that kind of fear alone.

"I'll protect you, Abigail," he said softly, meeting her gaze with unwavering resolve. "Whatever it takes, I'll make sure you and Sarah are safe."

She smiled, a flicker of warmth breaking through the fatigue. "Thank you, James. It means more than I can say."

Just then, the door creaked open, and Sarah peeked out, her wide eyes studying James with a mixture of curiosity and caution. She was a small, quiet child, but in her mother's presence, she was already learning to be brave.

"Momma, are you all right?" she asked, her voice barely more than a whisper.

Abigail turned and knelt, gathering her daughter in her arms. "Yes, sweetheart. Deputy Hamilton's here to help us."

Sarah glanced shyly at James, her grip on her mother tightening. He offered her a gentle smile, trying to ease her fears. "Don't worry, Sarah. I'm here to make sure nothing bad happens to you or your mom."

The girl managed a small nod, but her gaze was still clouded with uncertainty. James couldn't blame her—Jones's men had made sure that fear was a part of her young life, and that thought alone strengthened his resolve.

Abigail rose, guiding Sarah back inside with a reassuring smile. Then she turned back to James, her face clouded with worry. "They've been coming by at all hours," she said quietly. "They know where to find me when you're not around. They make threats…about the land, about what might happen if we don't leave."

A surge of anger rose within him, but he kept his voice calm. "Has anyone tried to come inside? Or lay a hand on either of you?"

"No," she replied, though her voice wavered. "But they make it clear that it's only a matter of time."

James nodded, already forming a plan in his mind. "I'll make sure there's someone keeping watch here when I can't be. And if you hear anything—any noise or anyone near the property—signal me. I'll be here as fast as I can."

Abigail's face softened with gratitude, but beneath it, he could see a flicker of guilt. "I don't want to put you in danger, James. You've already done so much."

He shook his head firmly. "It's not just about you, Abigail. It's about every homesteader and rancher trying to make a life here. Jones has to understand that he doesn't control everything. And he will, if we stand up to him together."

Abigail took a shaky breath, her shoulders straightening. "Then that's what we'll do."

For a moment, they shared a look of quiet understanding, the weight of their burdens momentarily lightened by the knowledge that they didn't have to carry them alone. She was a strong woman, but even the strongest needed someone to lean on every now and then.

"Thank you, James," she murmured, her eyes lingering on his. "Not just for us, but for everyone here."

He nodded, touched by her sincerity. "It's the right thing to do, Abigail. That's reason enough."

She gave a small smile, and for the first time in days, he saw a glimmer of hope in her eyes. It was a reminder of why he'd taken up the badge—to give people like her a chance at a life free from fear.

As he mounted his horse to leave, he gave her one last nod. "I'll be back to check on you soon. If anything happens, don't hesitate to send word."

She nodded, watching him with a steady gaze. "We'll be here, and we'll be ready."

As he rode away, the weight of his promise settled firmly on his shoulders. Abigail's plight was more than just her own; it was a battle for the soul of Sagebrush itself. For too long, people had lived under the shadow of men like Jones, believing that no one would stand up to them. But he was determined to show them that the law could still mean something.

His mind wandered back to Abigail and Sarah as he rode, the image of them standing on that porch etched in his memory. He thought of his own family, lost to violence and greed, and a wave of fierce determination washed over him.

This time, things would be different. This time, he wouldn't lose.

As he made his way back toward town, the setting sun bathed the plains in a golden light, casting long shadows across the land. It was a reminder of the darkness that hovered over them all, but also a symbol of the light that could drive it away.

With Abigail and the other settlers beside him, he knew they stood a chance. And with every mile he rode, he felt the weight of his mission settle into place, solid and unbreakable.

Whatever it took, he would see this through.

6. Ambush in the Hills

The sun was beginning to dip below the horizon, casting long shadows across the rolling hills as James Hamilton rode through the rugged terrain outside of Sagebrush. He had taken to the hills for his patrol, the elevation giving him a vantage point to watch for any trouble that might be brewing. With every mile, he felt the tension in the air grow thicker, as though the very land was holding its breath, waiting for something to happen.

He rode quietly, the rhythmic sound of hooves on dirt blending with the chirping of crickets and the soft rustle of leaves in the breeze. The solitude of the hills was a welcome reprieve from the tension of town, where he felt the weight of his promise to

Abigail and the settlers pressing down on him. But as much as he needed this moment of peace, he couldn't shake the feeling that something was off.

As he rounded a bend, a distant sound pierced the stillness—a series of galloping hooves, echoing through the valley. James immediately tensed, his instincts kicking in. He pulled his horse to a stop, scanning the area for signs of movement. His heart raced as he strained to hear over the thumping of his pulse.

It didn't take long for his fears to be confirmed. A group of men appeared over the crest of the hill, riding hard and fast. At the front was Clayton Yates, one of Jones's most ruthless enforcers. Yates was known for his cold demeanor and quick temper, a man who had little regard for anyone who stood in Jones's way.

"Looks like we've got ourselves a little lawman out here," Yates called out, his voice dripping with mockery. The men behind him laughed, the sound harsh and taunting as they circled James, cutting off any chance of escape.

James didn't flinch, keeping his grip steady on the reins. He had been expecting trouble from Jones's men, but he hadn't anticipated an ambush. He quickly calculated his options, weighing the odds of fighting versus fleeing.

"Yates," he said evenly, forcing himself to maintain a calm demeanor. "What do you want?"

Yates dismounted with a flourish, a sly grin spreading across his face. "What do I want?

Well, let's see... Jones wants your pretty little badge, and I'm here to collect. You've been a thorn in our side long enough."

James's heart pounded in his chest, but he refused to show any signs of fear. "You think you can just take it from me? You think this is some kind of game?"

The laughter from Yates's men grew louder, and James felt a surge of anger. He had made a promise to protect the people of this land, and he wasn't about to let these thugs intimidate him.

"No games, Deputy," Yates replied, taking a step closer. "Just a little lesson in respect. You're outnumbered, and this is our territory now. It'd be wise to back off while you can."

James's mind raced as he assessed the situation. He could see that Yates's men were eager for a fight, their hands resting on their weapons, eyes glinting with malicious intent. But he also knew he had the element of surprise on his side.

Without warning, Yates lunged forward, his fist raised. James instinctively sidestepped, ducking beneath Yates's swing and pivoting to put distance between them. He drew his gun, aiming it at Yates, who staggered back in shock.

The men behind Yates reacted quickly, drawing their guns as James took aim. "I suggest you think carefully about your next move," he warned, keeping his eyes locked on Yates. "This isn't the first time I've dealt with men like you."

Yates's bravado faltered momentarily, but he quickly regained his composure, raising his hands in mock surrender. "Is that a threat,

Deputy? Because if it is, I'd say you're outgunned."

Before James could respond, the sound of galloping hooves echoed through the valley again, but this time it was accompanied by a sudden rush of air as several of Yates's men charged him from the sides.

In a split second, James made a choice. He dove to the ground, rolling to avoid the hail of bullets that erupted around him. He felt the wind of a bullet pass close to his ear, the realization of how quickly the tide could turn crashing down on him.

He scrambled to his feet, searching for cover. A cluster of boulders lay nearby, and he sprinted toward them, his heart racing as he sought refuge. He ducked behind the rocks just as another barrage of gunfire erupted, bullets ricocheting off the stone and sending dust and debris flying.

"Don't let him get away!" Yates shouted, his voice laced with fury. "Surround him!"

James took a deep breath, his mind racing. He could hear the men closing in, their footsteps heavy on the ground. He knew he needed to act quickly before they closed off all avenues of escape.

He peered around the boulder, spotting a small rise in the terrain ahead. If he could make it to the top, he could use the elevation to his advantage. He took a moment to steady himself, then sprinted toward the rise, dodging behind the rocks for cover.

As he reached the top, he quickly scanned the area, looking for Yates and his men. They were scrambling, their attention focused on the boulders below, unaware of his new position. With a steadying breath, James took aim, his sharpshooting instincts kicking in as he prepared to fire.

He picked off one of Yates's men with a precise shot, the man falling to the ground in a flurry of dust. The other men reacted immediately, shouting in panic as they realized what was happening.

"Fall back!" Yates barked, his voice cutting through the chaos. "Get out of here!"

James took advantage of the confusion, firing off another shot that struck another man in the shoulder, causing him to go down with a cry. Yates, realizing the tide had turned, scrambled to mount his horse, his face twisted in anger and fear.

"Don't think this is over, Hamilton!" he shouted, spurring his horse away from the scene. "We'll settle this another day!"

James watched as the remaining men retreated, scrambling to regroup and escape the onslaught of his gunfire. His heart pounded in his chest, adrenaline coursing through him as he took a moment to catch his breath. He had narrowly escaped a dangerous situation, but he knew this wouldn't be the last encounter with Jones's men.

With the immediate threat gone, James took a moment to assess the area, his senses still heightened. He scanned for any remaining danger before cautiously making his way down the rise, returning to the path where he had first encountered the ambush.

As he rode away from the hills, his mind raced with thoughts of Abigail and the others. This skirmish was just a taste of the danger that lay ahead. Charles Jones wouldn't stop until he got what he wanted, and it was clear that James was firmly in his sights.

The sun dipped below the horizon, casting a fiery glow across the sky, but even its warmth couldn't quell the unease that settled over him. The battle for Sagebrush was only just beginning, and James knew he needed to rally the settlers—Abigail and her daughter, Hank, and anyone else willing to stand up against Jones.

He wouldn't let fear dictate their futures any longer. They would fight back, and together, they would reclaim their land and their lives.

7. The Homesteaders Revolt

The meeting hall in Sagebrush was bustling with murmurs as James Hamilton stepped inside. The wooden structure, usually filled with the laughter and chatter of townsfolk, was now cloaked in a heavy atmosphere of worry and determination. Farmers, ranchers, and their families filled the benches, casting anxious glances toward the front where James stood, ready to address the crowd.

"Thank you all for coming," James began, his voice cutting through the din of conversation. "I know times are tough, and I know many of you are scared. But if we're going to protect our homes, we need to come together."

As he spoke, he scanned the faces before him. Abigail Kennedy sat near the front, her expression resolute, while Charles Jones's threats loomed large in the minds of those gathered. He could see the fear in their eyes, but beneath it flickered a spark of defiance. They were tired of being bullied, tired of living under the shadow of Jones's tyranny.

"We all know that Charles Jones and his men won't stop until they've taken what they want," he continued, pacing before the assembly. "They've already tried to intimidate us, to push us off our land. But we can't let them win. We have the right to our homes, our lives, and we need to fight for them."

A low murmur rippled through the crowd, a mix of uncertainty and growing determination. James could feel the tension shift, the air crackling with the potential for change. He pressed on, driven by a fierce resolve to inspire action.

"Together, we're stronger," he urged. "I'm asking each of you to join me. Let's fortify our homes, set up patrols, and be prepared to stand our ground. We need to show Jones that we're not afraid to fight back."

Abigail stood, her voice steady and clear. "James is right. I've faced his men alone, and I can tell you—it's terrifying. But if we stand together, we can protect what's ours. We can't let them take our land, our families, our futures!"

Nods of agreement rippled through the crowd, and James felt a surge of hope. They needed to harness that determination, to turn it into action.

"We'll need to work quickly," James said, outlining a plan. "Let's divide into groups. We can start reinforcing our fences, setting up lookouts, and preparing to defend our land. We have the advantage of knowing these hills, the terrain. We can use that to our benefit."

The crowd erupted into excited chatter, a mix of fear and resolve igniting a fire within them. Farmers discussed their properties, strategizing ways to fortify their defenses while ranchers shared stories of past conflicts, each tale fueling the collective anger toward Jones's tyranny.

Over the next hour, the mood shifted from uncertainty to determination. They broke into smaller groups, discussing specific strategies. James moved from one group to another, offering guidance, encouragement, and a steady presence as they organized their defenses.

By the end of the meeting, James felt a renewed sense of purpose among the homesteaders. They were no longer just a collection of frightened individuals; they had become a united front. It was a powerful shift, and he could sense the fear beginning to dissipate, replaced by a resolve to protect what was rightfully theirs.

As the sun began to set, painting the sky in hues of orange and red, the homesteaders dispersed, energized by their newfound purpose. James stood at the door, watching them go, knowing that this was only the beginning.

"Thank you, James," Abigail said, stepping up beside him. Her voice was laced with admiration and gratitude. "You've inspired them to fight."

He shrugged modestly, feeling the weight of responsibility settle on his shoulders. "They're the ones who showed courage. All I did was give them a reason to believe in themselves."

"Still, you made them believe they could fight back," she replied, her eyes shining with respect. "You've given us hope."

As darkness enveloped the town, James and Abigail discussed the next steps for their respective homesteads. They made plans for patrols, discussing who would be stationed where and how to communicate in case of an attack.

"Let's meet at my place tomorrow morning," Abigail suggested. "We can start reinforcing the fences and make sure everything is secure."

James nodded. "I'll bring the others. We'll need as many hands as we can get."

The two shared a moment of silence, the gravity of their situation settling over them. The bond they had forged in adversity was strong, and it gave him strength to face the challenges ahead.

"Are you sure you're ready for this?" James asked, his tone turning serious. "I know it's going to get dangerous."

Abigail's expression shifted, determination hardening her features. "I've faced danger before, James. I won't back down now. Not for my daughter, not for this land."

Her fierce resolve stirred something deep within him. It reminded him that their fight wasn't just about land; it was about families, futures, and the right to live free from fear.

As they parted ways, James couldn't shake the feeling that they were on the precipice of something monumental. The homesteaders were no longer victims; they were fighters, ready to stand up for their rights.

The next morning, the sun rose to find the homesteaders gathered at Abigail's place, ready to begin fortifying the land. Armed with tools, determination, and a sense of purpose, they began working together to strengthen their defenses.

James moved among them, directing traffic, offering advice, and encouraging the men and women as they worked. Each time he caught a glimpse of Abigail, sweat glistening on her brow as she directed her daughter to help haul supplies, he felt a swell of admiration.

"Let's get these fences reinforced!" he shouted, rallying the group as they worked. "We need to make it clear to Jones and his men that this land is ours!"

As the sun climbed higher, the homesteaders moved with purpose, reinforcing fences, creating makeshift barriers, and scouting the surrounding hills for any signs of trouble. The sense of camaraderie and determination among them grew with each passing hour, and James felt a surge of pride at the sight of their unity.

But deep in his gut, the tension lingered. He knew that Jones wouldn't take their defiance lightly. The cattle baron was used to getting what he wanted, and the revolt of the homesteaders would surely provoke a response.

As evening fell, the group gathered once more, exhausted but triumphant. They had made significant progress, but James couldn't shake the feeling that they were still on borrowed time. Jones wouldn't let this stand, and he would come for them.

"Keep your eyes open tonight," James urged as they prepared to head home. "We may not have seen the last of Jones and his men."

As they dispersed into the shadows of the evening, James couldn't help but feel a sense of foreboding settle over him. The battle for their lives and homes had only just begun, and he would do everything in his power to protect them.

With Abigail and the homesteaders behind him, he steeled himself for the confrontation ahead. Together, they would fight for their land, their families, and their future. And he would ensure that they wouldn't have to face this battle alone.

8. The Battle of Lost Canyon

The air was thick with tension as dawn broke over Lost Canyon, illuminating the rugged cliffs and the narrow passage that would soon become a battleground. James Hamilton stood at the mouth of the canyon, surveying the landscape with a steely gaze. He could feel the weight of the moment pressing down on him; today would determine the future of Sagebrush and the homesteaders who had put their faith in him.

The plan was simple but risky. James had chosen Lost Canyon for its natural defenses—its steep walls and narrow entry points would work in their favor. With the homesteaders set to defend the canyon, he hoped they could outmaneuver Charles

Jones and his men, using strategy and determination to offset their numerical disadvantage.

As the sun climbed higher in the sky, the homesteaders began to assemble, their faces a mix of fear and resolve. Abigail was among them, her expression fierce as she tightened her grip on her rifle. James felt a swell of admiration for her bravery; she was a force to be reckoned with, ready to stand and fight for her daughter and her land.

"Listen up!" James called out, gathering the attention of the assembled group. "Today, we stand together against a man who thinks he can take what is ours. Remember, we're fighting for our homes, our families, and our way of life. If we stick to the plan and support each other, we can drive them out.

We're not just defending this canyon; we're defending our future."

Nods of agreement rippled through the crowd, and James could see the resolve building among the homesteaders. He glanced at Abigail, who stood tall, her determination unshakeable. He knew that they would give their all, and he intended to lead them to victory.

As the sounds of hoofbeats echoed in the distance, a hush fell over the group. James turned to see the dust rising in the air, signaling the approach of Jones's men. He could make out the silhouette of Charles Jones at the front, his arrogance unmistakable as he rode confidently into the canyon.

"Remember our plan!" James called out, positioning the homesteaders along the rocky walls, ensuring they had clear lines of sight and cover. "Stay low and be ready to move. We'll catch them off guard!"

The tension crackled in the air as Jones's men entered the canyon, their shouts echoing off the walls. "Come out, come out, wherever you are!" Jones taunted, a cruel grin plastered across his face. "You think you can hide from us?"

James's heart raced. It was time. "Now!" he shouted, signaling the homesteaders to open fire.

A barrage of gunfire erupted from the walls of the canyon, echoing like thunder as bullets whizzed through the air. James aimed carefully, picking off one of Jones's men with a precise shot. The chaos of battle unfolded around him—cries of determination mingled with the shouts of

Jones's men, who were caught off guard by the ferocity of the homesteaders' defense.

James moved swiftly along the rocky terrain, rallying the settlers and directing their fire. "Focus on their horses! If we can't let them regroup, we can gain the upper hand!" He watched as the homesteaders followed his lead, targeting the mounts, causing panic among Jones's ranks.

The battle was fierce, with dust swirling and the sound of gunfire drowning out everything else. But James felt a rush of adrenaline as he witnessed the spirit of the homesteaders; they fought with the desperation and determination of those who had everything to lose.

Amid the chaos, Abigail fought valiantly alongside her neighbors, her eyes focused and unyielding. James admired her bravery as she moved with purpose, supporting those around her. They were a team now, fighting for their land and their families, united against the threat posed by Jones.

Suddenly, James spotted Jones himself in the fray, barking orders to his men. He was furious, his face twisted in rage as he realized the tide of the battle was turning against him. James took a deep breath, steeling himself for what was to come.

He made his way through the chaos, weaving between the rocks, eyes locked on Jones. This confrontation was personal—Jones had underestimated him, and now he would pay the price. As he approached, James felt the adrenaline surge through him, fueling his resolve.

"James Hamilton!" Jones shouted, his voice rising above the din. "You're a fool to think you can stand against me! I'll bury you in this canyon!"

With a fierce determination, James drew his gun and faced Jones directly. "You won't take this land, Jones. Not while I'm alive to stop you!"

The two men stood locked in a tense standoff, the noise of the battle fading into the background as they squared off. James's heart pounded in his chest as he took aim, the world around him blurring into insignificance.

Just as Jones reached for his weapon, a gunshot rang out from one of his men, sending James diving for cover. Bullets flew overhead, and chaos erupted anew as Jones's men regrouped, their morale bolstered by their leader's presence.

"Regroup! Flank them from the sides!" Jones commanded, his voice booming with authority. James knew he had to act quickly to regain control of the situation.

"Stay together!" he shouted to the homesteaders. "We can't let them split us up! Hold your ground!"

With renewed focus, James rallied the homesteaders, encouraging them to push back against Jones's forces. They took advantage of the rocky terrain, using it for cover as they exchanged fire with the cattlemen. The tide began to shift as the homesteaders found their footing, their determination amplifying their resolve.

"Move! Move!" James yelled, leading a charge toward Jones's men. The homesteaders surged forward, fueled by the fire of their purpose. They were no longer just defending; they were fighting back.

James caught sight of Abigail, firing with precision as she supported the others. "Keep pushing forward!" he called to her, his voice steady despite the chaos around them. "We can't let them regroup!"

The fierce exchange continued, the sounds of gunfire and shouting filling the canyon. It felt like an eternity, but inch by inch, the homesteaders gained ground. They pressed against Jones's men, who began to falter under the relentless assault.

Then, as the battle reached its peak, James spotted an opening. He took a deep breath, his mind racing with strategy, and quickly formed a plan. "We're going to flank them from the right!" he shouted to Abigail and the others. "Follow me!"

With adrenaline coursing through him, James led the charge, maneuvering around the rocky outcrops. They moved in a tight formation, closing in on Jones's men from the side. The surprise attack caught them off guard, and James felt a rush of triumph as they began to break through.

The sounds of battle shifted from chaos to desperation as Jones's men realized they were surrounded. James could see the panic in their eyes as they turned to flee, their bravado crumbling under the pressure of the homesteaders' relentless pursuit.

"Don't let them escape!" James called out, his voice rising above the din. "This is our chance!"

With a final push, the homesteaders surged forward, their resolve solidifying as they drove Jones's men deeper into the canyon.

The sound of hooves and shouts echoed off the cliffs, but the tide of the battle had shifted. They were winning.

As the last remnants of Jones's forces retreated, James stood tall, breathing heavily as he surveyed the scene. The canyon was now theirs, a hard-won victory etched into the very ground beneath their feet.

The homesteaders erupted into cheers, their voices rising in celebration. James felt a sense of pride swell within him. They had come together, united in purpose, and driven out a man who had sought to destroy their lives.

Abigail stood beside him, her face flushed with exhilaration. "We did it, James! We actually did it!" she exclaimed, her eyes sparkling with triumph.

James smiled, the weight of the moment settling over him. "We fought for what's right. This victory belongs to all of us."

As the dust settled and the sounds of battle faded, the homesteaders gathered, their spirits lifted. Together, they had faced a formidable foe and emerged victorious, their bond forged in the fires of conflict.

But as James stood among them, he couldn't shake the feeling that this battle was just the beginning. Charles Jones would not take his defeat lightly, and they would need to remain vigilant.

The sun dipped lower in the sky, but James knew that the light of their victory would guide them forward. They had proven they could stand together, and now they would face whatever challenges lay ahead with courage and determination. The fight for their land and their future was far from over, but they were ready to face it, united as one.

9. Charles Jones's Last Stand

The night after the battle in Lost Canyon was eerily quiet, a stark contrast to the chaos and gunfire that had filled the air just hours earlier. James Hamilton stood watch outside Abigail Kennedy's homestead, the cool breeze whispering through the trees, a reminder that while the day had brought them victory, the threat of Charles Jones was far from over.

As the stars glittered in the vast night sky, James felt a sense of unease creeping over him. He had fought hard alongside the homesteaders, but he knew that a man like Jones would not easily accept defeat. The cattle baron was cornered now, desperate and humiliated, and such men often resorted to the most dangerous measures when they felt threatened.

"James," Abigail's voice broke the stillness as she approached him, her silhouette illuminated by the soft glow of the moonlight. "Are you sure it's wise to be out here alone?"

He turned to face her, a reassuring smile on his lips. "I'll be fine, Abigail. I just want to make sure everything is secure. Jones won't rest until he's had his revenge."

Abigail nodded, her brow furrowing with concern. "I just worry that he'll come after you. He won't take this loss lightly."

"I know," James replied, his gaze drifting toward the dark horizon. "But we need to be prepared for whatever he might try. We can't let our guard down."

Just then, a distant rumble of thunder echoed across the sky, a reminder of the storm brewing on the horizon—both in the weather and in the brewing conflict with Jones. As James scanned the area, he felt an unsettling tension, as if the very air was charged with anticipation.

Back at the ranch, the remaining homesteaders were beginning to rest after the day's exertions, and Abigail's daughter, who had fallen asleep earlier, lay safe in her bed. But James couldn't shake the feeling that something was coming, something dangerous.

Hours passed, and just as the first drops of rain began to fall, a sound broke the quiet—hooves pounding against the ground. James's heart raced as he reached for his rifle, eyes narrowing as he scanned the path leading toward the homestead. He knew that sound all too well; it was the unmistakable approach of men on horseback.

"Stay inside, Abigail," he ordered, his voice firm. "Lock the door and keep your daughter safe."

With a quick nod, Abigail slipped back into the house, and James positioned himself behind a tree, waiting for the riders to emerge from the shadows. As the figures approached, he recognized the familiar silhouette of Charles Jones, flanked by several of his most loyal men, all armed and ready for a fight.

"Come out, Hamilton!" Jones's voice boomed across the clearing, laced with venomous fury. "I know you're out there, you coward! Face me like a man!"

James clenched his jaw, his grip tightening around the rifle. Jones was a dangerous man, but his desperation made him even more unpredictable. "I'm not afraid of you, Jones!" he shouted back, stepping into view, the rain now falling steadily around him. "You've already lost. Leave this place, and we won't have any more trouble."

"Trouble?" Jones laughed bitterly, his voice echoing in the stillness of the night. "You think you can tell me what to do? You've humiliated me in front of my men! You've taken my land, my power, and now you'll pay the price!"

With that, Jones motioned to his men, and they surged forward, weapons drawn. James knew he had only moments to act. He fired a shot, striking one of Jones's men and sending the others scattering for cover. The night erupted into chaos as gunfire rang out, the air thick with the smell of gunpowder and the sound of hooves pounding the muddy ground.

"Get him!" Jones shouted, his voice filled with rage as he charged toward James, a gun drawn and aimed directly at him.

James ducked behind a nearby tree, narrowly avoiding a volley of bullets. The rain began to pour, soaking him to the bone, but he didn't hesitate. He could hear the sound of Jones's men regrouping, and he knew that time was running out.

"Jones, this ends now!" James shouted, his voice steady despite the chaos surrounding him. "You can't win this fight! You've lost everything!"

"Lost everything?" Jones bellowed, fury twisting his features. "I'll show you what it means to lose, Hamilton!"

With a sudden surge of adrenaline, James burst from his cover, aiming carefully as he moved through the rain-soaked terrain. He could see Jones now, his expression twisted with hatred, and he took a deep breath, focusing on his target.

In a fierce exchange of gunfire, James ducked and dodged, using the trees for cover as he closed in on his enemy. The rain poured down in sheets, making the ground slick and treacherous, but he pressed on, driven by a sense of justice that burned fiercely within him.

Just as James rounded a thick oak tree, he spotted Jones preparing to fire at him. In that split second, he realized that this was it—the moment he had been waiting for. With his heart pounding in his chest, he steadied his aim and fired, striking Jones in the shoulder.

The cattle baron stumbled back, a look of shock crossing his face as he clutched the wound. "You...you'll pay for this, Hamilton!" he spat, his voice strained with pain and fury.

James didn't relent; he advanced, his expression firm. "You're finished, Jones. It's time to answer for your crimes."

With a final surge of determination, James disarmed Jones, knocking the gun from his hand and pinning him against a nearby tree. The rain continued to pour, mixing with the blood that stained the ground beneath them.

"You think you can intimidate us?" James said, his voice low and fierce. "You think you can bully people off their land? Not anymore."

The other men, witnessing their leader's defeat, began to hesitate, exchanging uncertain glances. James turned slightly, addressing them. "It's over! You can either join us in building a better community or continue following a man who's lost everything. Make your choice!"

One by one, the men began to lower their weapons, stepping back from the fight. Jones, now desperate and cornered, glared at his men, but the resolve in their eyes was unmistakable. They were no longer willing to fight for a man who had led them to this point of ruin.

"Marshal Jackson will be here soon," James warned, tightening his grip on Jones.

"You're going to stand trial for what you've done."

Jones's eyes darkened with rage as he struggled against James's grip. "You think you can keep me here? You're making a mistake, Hamilton. I won't go down without a fight!"

"Then you'll find yourself fighting against the law," James replied, his voice unwavering. "You're done here."

As the sounds of hoofbeats echoed in the distance, James knew that Marshal Jackson would soon arrive to take Jones into custody. The tension in the air began to dissipate, replaced by a sense of triumph and relief.

"Let's get him out of here," James ordered, motioning for the remaining homesteaders to step forward and assist in securing Jones.

They moved with purpose, binding his hands and leading him away from the scene of his defeat.

As they made their way back toward the homestead, the rain began to lighten, and the clouds parted, revealing a sliver of moonlight. James felt a weight lift from his shoulders as he led Jones away, knowing that they had finally triumphed over the tyranny that had plagued their lives.

When they reached the homestead, Marshal Jackson was waiting, a stern expression on his face. "What's going on here?" he asked, taking in the sight of Jones being led in shackles.

"James Hamilton," James replied, meeting Jackson's gaze with determination. "We've captured Charles Jones. He's ready to stand trial for his crimes."

Jackson nodded, a flicker of respect crossing his features. "Good work, Hamilton. It's about time we put an end to this."

With that, the homesteaders watched as Marshal Jackson took custody of Jones, the cattle baron's fate now in the hands of the law. As he was led away, James felt a surge of satisfaction, knowing that they had not only defended their homes but also brought justice to a man who had tried to destroy them.

In the days that followed, the homesteaders began to rebuild and reclaim their lives. The storm had passed, leaving behind a clearer sky and a renewed sense of hope. James had stood up to a powerful foe and emerged victorious, but more importantly, he had united a community that had once been fractured by fear.

As he walked alongside Abigail, watching the sun rise over the horizon, he felt a sense of peace settling within him. The battle was won, and together, they would build a brighter future.

James glanced at Abigail, who smiled softly at him, her eyes reflecting the light of the new day. They had faced adversity together and emerged stronger, united in their fight for justice and their land.

"Thank you for everything, James," she said, her voice sincere. "You've changed our lives."

"We did this together," he replied, a smile breaking through his serious demeanor. "And we'll keep fighting for what's right."

As the sun climbed higher, James knew that they had forged a new path, one filled with possibilities. They had stood together against the darkness and emerged victorious, ready to face whatever challenges lay ahead, united in hope and strength.

10. A New Beginning

The sun rose over the town of Sagebrush, casting a warm golden hue across the landscape. The remnants of the storm that had passed through a few days earlier were gone, leaving behind a refreshed world filled with hope. The townsfolk moved about with a renewed energy, their spirits lifted now that the threat of Charles Jones had been vanquished.

James Hamilton stood on the porch of Abigail Kennedy's homestead, watching as the community gathered in the clearing nearby. Homesteaders exchanged stories, laughter echoing through the air as they worked together to repair the damage from the recent chaos. It was a sight that filled him with pride; they had come together as a united front, and now they were finally free to reclaim their lives.

Abigail approached him, her presence a balm to his weary soul. The soft breeze played with her hair, and for a moment, they stood together in silence, taking in the vibrant atmosphere around them.

"Looks like the town is starting to heal," James remarked, a smile tugging at his lips as he gestured toward the homesteaders working together.

Abigail returned his smile, her eyes shining with gratitude. "It's all thanks to you, James. You stood up to Jones when no one else would. You've given us hope again."

James felt a warmth spread through him at her words. "I couldn't have done it without everyone's support. We fought this battle together."

As they watched the scene unfold, a sense of tranquility settled over them. The laughter of children rang out, and the scent of fresh bread baking wafted through the air, reminding James of the simple joys that life could bring.

"Do you think it will stay like this?" Abigail asked, her tone thoughtful. "Will the peace last?"

James turned to her, his expression serious. "I believe it will. Jones is gone, and the people have finally found their voices. They won't let anyone push them around again."

Abigail nodded, though a flicker of uncertainty crossed her face. "I just hope that the fear he instilled in us doesn't linger too long."

"Fear is powerful, but so is hope," James said, reaching out to place a reassuring hand on her shoulder. "We've shown that we can stand together. That strength will carry us through."

Just then, the sound of hoofbeats approached, and they turned to see Marshal Wyatt Jackson riding up, a weary yet relieved look on his face. He dismounted and approached them, tipping his hat with a nod.

"James, Abigail," he greeted, his voice steady. "I wanted to thank you both for your roles in bringing Jones to justice. It wasn't an easy fight, but you did what had to be done."

James met Jackson's gaze, a sense of respect blossoming between them. "It was a community effort, Marshal. We all did our part."

"True enough," Jackson replied, glancing at the gathering crowd. "But your leadership made a significant difference. People look up to you, James. You've become a symbol of hope in these parts."

James felt the weight of those words. He had come to Sagebrush seeking to restore order, but in the process, he had found something much deeper—a sense of belonging and a connection to the land and its people.

As Jackson continued to speak, James's thoughts drifted back to Abigail. He could see the determination in her eyes, the resilience that had carried her through the darkest days. There was something special about their bond, and he knew that the journey they had taken together had only just begun.

"Abigail," James said, breaking away from the conversation with Jackson. "Can we talk for a moment?"

She looked at him, curiosity flickering in her eyes, and nodded. They moved a few paces away from the gathering crowd, the sounds of laughter and conversation fading into the background.

"What's on your mind?" Abigail asked, her voice soft but steady.

James took a deep breath, the weight of his feelings pressing against his chest. "I want you to know how much you mean to me, Abigail. Your strength and spirit have inspired me more than you can imagine."

A blush crept to Abigail's cheeks, but she held his gaze, unflinching. "You've been a beacon of hope for all of us, James. I've admired your courage and determination from the very beginning."

He stepped closer, feeling the electricity in the air between them. "I know the road ahead won't be easy. There will always be challenges, but I want to face them with you. I believe we can build something good here, together."

Her eyes widened in surprise, but then a smile broke through, illuminating her features. "You really mean that?"

"Absolutely," James replied, his heart racing. "I want to help you build a future for you and your daughter—a future where you can feel safe and thrive. If you'll let me, I'd like to be part of that future."

Abigail's expression softened, and she reached out to grasp his hand, her touch sending a surge of warmth through him. "I would like that very much, James. I've always wanted to believe that there was something more for us, something worth fighting for."

At that moment, James felt a sense of clarity wash over him. The challenges they had faced had forged a bond that was unbreakable, and together, they could overcome anything.

Suddenly, the laughter of the children drew their attention back to the crowd. The sight of them playing brought a smile to both their faces, a reminder of the innocence and joy they were fighting to protect.

"Before you go," Abigail said, her voice soft but filled with determination. "Promise me that you'll always look out for this community, for the homesteaders, and for us. We need someone like you to keep us safe."

James nodded, feeling the weight of her words settle in his heart. "I promise. As long as I'm here, I'll do everything I can to protect this land and its people."

"Good," she said, her smile brightening. "Because I believe in this place, and I believe in us."

As they stood together, hand in hand, the sun broke through the clouds, bathing them in warm light. It was a new beginning, not just for the town of Sagebrush but for James and Abigail as well.

After sharing a lingering look, James reluctantly pulled away, knowing he had to continue his work as a deputy. The town was just beginning to heal, and there was still much to do. "I'll see you soon, Abigail," he said, his voice filled with promise.

As he mounted his horse, James looked back at the homestead, where Abigail stood watching him, her daughter at her side. He rode away, knowing that he was not just a lawman in this territory but a protector of the hope and dreams that were beginning to flourish.

As he rode toward the horizon, the path ahead was filled with possibilities, and he knew that together with Abigail and the community, they would write a new chapter in their story—a story of resilience, unity, and hope. The promise of a brighter tomorrow shone brightly, waiting for them to claim it.

Other Books from Seniorality

To find your next book visit:
www.amazon.com/author/seniorality
Where you will find:

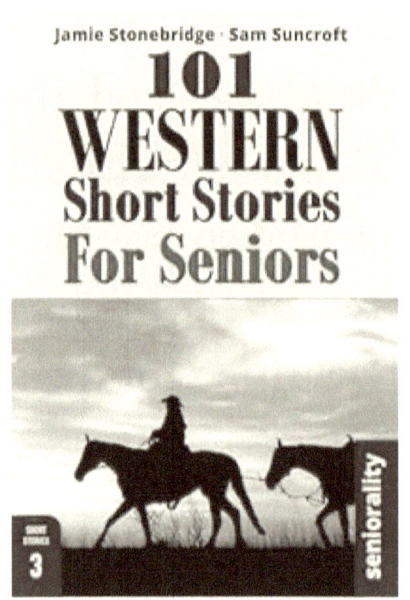 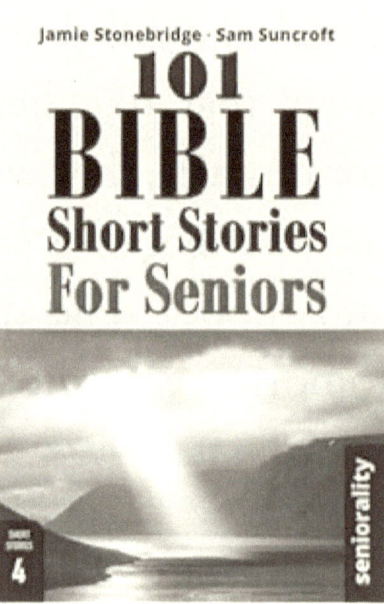

Short Stories

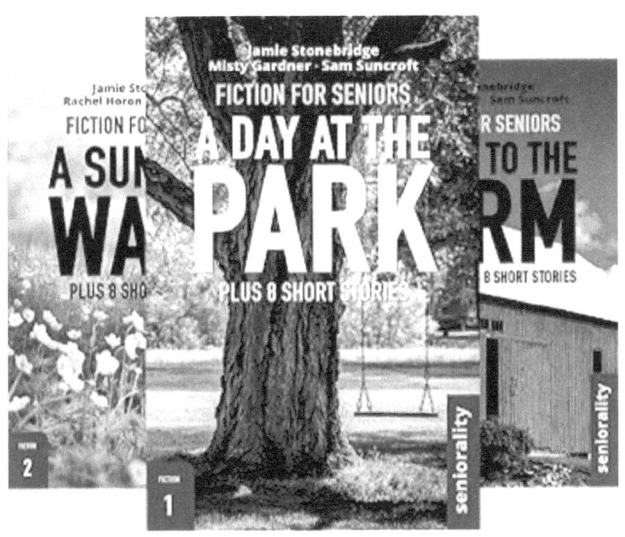

Fiction for Seniors

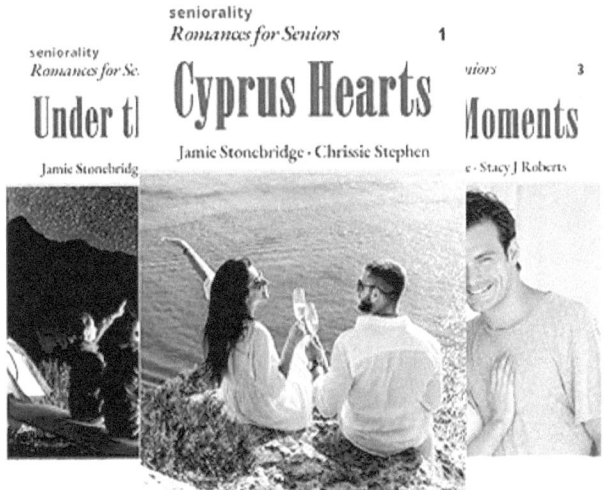

Romances for Seniors

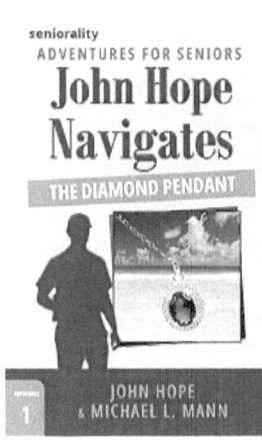 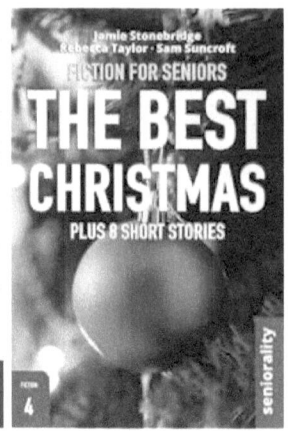 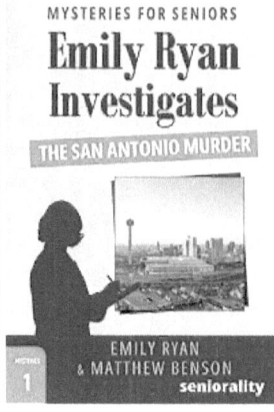

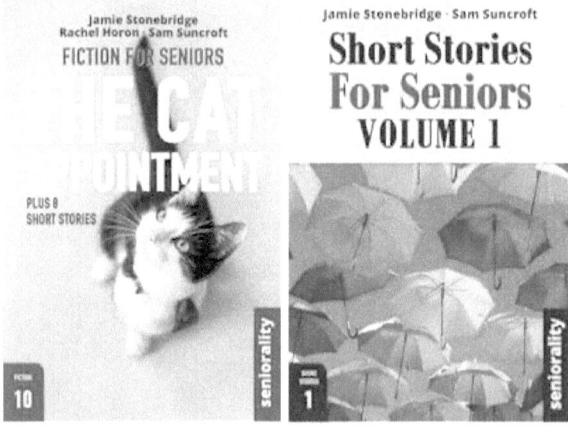

And More

Find these books by searching on Amazon for
'seniorality'

or visit:

www.amazon.com/author/seniorality

Thank You

If you enjoyed this book or found it useful, we'd be very grateful if you'd write a short review on Amazon.

Your support really does make a difference and helps other people discover this book.

We personally read all reviews to hear how the books are being used, to collect feedback, and get ideas for future stories.

Thank you and have a wonderful day!

www.ingramcontent.com/pod-product-compliance
Lightning Source LLC
Chambersburg PA
CBHW020439220526
45464CB00002B/774